THE SIBO DIET COOKBOOK FOR BEGINNERS

Easy, Delicious and Nutritious Recipes for Ideal Gut health

Jennifer Stewart

Table of contents

Introduction

"The SIBO Diet Cookbook for Beginners," is your go-to guide for embracing a diet that can make a significant difference in managing Small Intestinal Bacterial Overgrowth (SIBO). If you have been diagnosed with SIBO or suspect you might have it, you're in the right place. This cookbook aims to simplify the journey of adopting a diet tailored to support your gut health and overall well-being.

What is the SIBO Diet?

The SIBO diet is a therapeutic approach designed to manage the symptoms of Small Intestinal Bacterial Overgrowth, a condition characterized by an excessive amount of bacteria in the small intestine. These bacteria can ferment certain types of carbohydrates, leading to symptoms like bloating, gas, diarrhea, and abdominal pain. The primary goal of the SIBO diet is to reduce the intake of these fermentable carbohydrates, known as FODMAPs (Fermentable Oligosaccharides, Disaccharides, Monosaccharides, and Polyols), to alleviate digestive distress and improve gut health.

The Importance of Diet in Managing SIBO

Diet plays a crucial role in managing SIBO symptoms and promoting an optimal gut health. By eliminating or reducing the intake of FODMAP-rich foods that feed the bacteria causing the overgrowth, you can help restore balance in your gut and alleviate uncomfortable symptoms. Additionally, focusing on whole, nutrient-dense foods can support overall digestive function, enhance nutrient absorption, and boost your immune system.

Adopting a SIBO-friendly diet isn't just about what you eliminate but also about what you include. Incorporating a variety of vegetables, lean proteins, healthy fats, and gut-friendly foods like fermented vegetables and bone broth can provide essential nutrients and support a healthy microbiome.

Overview of the Cookbook

In "The SIBO Diet Cookbook for Beginners," you will ll find a collection of delicious and nutritious recipes designed specifically for those following the SIBO diet. From satisfying breakfasts and hearty mains to mouthwatering desserts and gut-healing beverages, this cookbook offers a diverse range of options to suit every taste and preference.

We'll start with a comprehensive introduction to SIBO, explaining what it is, its causes, symptoms, and treatment options. You'll learn about the benefits of the SIBO diet and why it's an essential part of managing this condition effectively.

Next, we'll guide you through getting started with the SIBO diet, including essential kitchen tools, pantry staples, and shopping tips to make meal planning a breeze. You'll also discover SIBO-friendly cooking techniques to help you create flavorful and satisfying meals without compromising on taste.

The heart of this cookbook lies in its diverse range of recipes, carefully crafted to be delicious, easy to prepare, and compliant with the SIBO diet guidelines. Each recipe comes with detailed instructions, nutritional information, and modification options to cater to various dietary needs and preferences.

Whether you're new to the SIBO diet or looking for fresh inspiration to spice up your meals, "The SIBO Diet Cookbook for Beginners" is your ultimate resource for embracing a diet that supports your gut health and helps you live your best life.

Chapter 1:

Understanding SIBO

What is SIBO?

Small Intestinal Bacterial Overgrowth, or SIBO, is a condition characterized by an excessive amount of bacteria in the small intestine. Normally, the small intestine contains relatively few bacteria compared to the large intestine. However, when there's an overgrowth of bacteria in the small intestine, it can lead to various digestive symptoms and discomfort.

These bacteria can ferment certain types of carbohydrates, producing gases like hydrogen and methane, which can cause symptoms such as bloating, gas, diarrhea, abdominal pain, and even malabsorption of nutrients. Managing

SIBO often involves dietary changes, as well as other treatment approaches, to help restore balance in the gut and alleviate symptoms.

Causes and Symptoms

The exact cause of SIBO can vary from person to person, but some common factors include:

- **Impaired Gut Motility**: Conditions that affect the movement of the small intestine, such as irritable bowel syndrome (IBS) or surgery, can contribute to SIBO.
- **Low Stomach Acid:** Reduced stomach acid levels can allow bacteria to proliferate in the small intestine.
- **Anatomical Abnormalities:** Structural issues in the digestive tract, like strictures or fistulas, can lead to bacterial overgrowth.

- **Medications**: Certain medications, such as proton pump inhibitors (PPIs) or antibiotics, can disrupt the balance of bacteria in the gut and contribute to SIBO.

As for symptoms, they can vary widely but commonly include:
- Bloating and abdominal distension,
- Gas and flatulence,
- Diarrhea or constipation,
- Abdominal pain or cramping,
- Fatigue and weakness,
- Nutritional deficiencies due to malabsorption.

It's essential to note that SIBO symptoms can overlap with other gastrointestinal conditions, making diagnosis challenging. If you're experiencing persistent digestive issues, it's crucial to consult with a healthcare professional for an accurate diagnosis and appropriate treatment plan.

Diagnosis and Treatment Options .

Diagnosing SIBO typically involves a combination of clinical evaluation, symptom assessment, and specific tests. Some common diagnostic tests for SIBO include:

1. **Breath Tests:** These tests measure the levels of hydrogen and methane gasses produced by bacteria in the small intestine after consuming a substrate like lactulose or glucose.
2. **Small Intestine Aspirate:** In some cases, a sample of fluid from the small intestine may be collected and analyzed to identify bacterial overgrowth directly.
3. **Blood Tests:** These can help identify underlying conditions or nutritional deficiencies associated with SIBO.

Once diagnosed, treatment for SIBO often focuses on:

1. Dietary Changes: Adopting a SIBO-friendly diet low in fermentable carbohydrates (FODMAPs) can help manage symptoms and reduce bacterial overgrowth.
2. Antibiotics: Depending on the severity of SIBO, your healthcare provider may prescribe antibiotics to reduce bacterial overgrowth in the small intestine.
3. Probiotics and Gut Health Support: Probiotics and other gut-supporting supplements can help restore balance to the gut microbiome and promote overall digestive health.

In this cookbook, we'll focus on the dietary aspect of managing SIBO, offering you a variety of delicious and nutritious recipes designed to support your gut health and alleviate symptoms.

As always, it's essential to work closely with your healthcare provider to develop a comprehensive treatment plan tailored to your individual needs.

Chapter 2:

Benefits of the SIBO Diet

While managing SIBO can be challenging, making informed dietary choices can significantly improve your digestive health, enhance nutrient absorption, and effectively manage SIBO symptoms. Let's explore these benefits in detail.

1. Improving Digestive Health

One of the primary goals of the SIBO diet is to restore balance to your gut microbiome by reducing the overgrowth of bacteria in the small intestine. By eliminating or reducing the intake of fermentable carbohydrates, known as FODMAPs, you can help alleviate digestive distress and create a more hospitable environment for beneficial gut bacteria.

A balanced and healthy gut microbiome is essential for optimal digestive function. It helps break down food, absorb nutrients, regulate bowel movements, and support overall gut health. By following a SIBO-friendly diet, you can promote a healthier gut environment, reduce inflammation, and improve overall digestive comfort.

2. Enhancing Nutrient Absorption.

SIBO can interfere with the absorption of essential nutrients, leading to deficiencies and various health issues. The overgrowth of bacteria in the small intestine can impair the integrity of the intestinal lining, reducing its ability to absorb nutrients effectively.

A SIBO-friendly diet focuses on nutrient-dense, whole foods that are easier to digest and absorb, such as lean proteins, non-starchy vegetables, and healthy fats. By choosing foods that are less likely to cause digestive upset and malabsorption, you can enhance your body's ability to absorb essential vitamins, minerals, and other nutrients, supporting overall health and well-being.

Managing SIBO Symptoms

One of the most compelling benefits of the SIBO diet is its ability to manage and alleviate the uncomfortable symptoms associated with SIBO, such as bloating, gas, diarrhea, and abdominal pain. By reducing the intake of fermentable carbohydrates that feed the bacteria causing the overgrowth, you can significantly reduce gas production and bloating.

Moreover, by focusing on gut-friendly foods and avoiding triggers that exacerbate symptoms, you can create a meal plan that supports digestive comfort and helps manage SIBO symptoms effectively. Incorporating anti-inflammatory foods, gut-healing ingredients, and digestive aids can further enhance symptom relief and promote overall gut health.

In summary, adopting a SIBO-friendly diet offers a holistic approach to managing SIBO by improving digestive health, enhancing nutrient absorption, and effectively managing symptoms. As you explore the recipes and meal plans in this cookbook, you'll discover how easy and delicious it can be to eat for gut health, supporting your journey towards optimal well-being.

Chapter 3:

Getting Started with the SIBO Diet.

Kitchen Tools and Equipment

Having the right kitchen tools and equipment can make meal preparation a breeze and help you create delicious SIBO-friendly meals with ease. Here are some essential items you'll want to have on hand:

1. **High-Quality Chef's Knife:** A sharp chef's knife is essential for chopping, slicing, and dicing fruits, vegetables, and proteins.
2. **Cutting Board:** Opt for a durable cutting board made of wood or plastic that's easy to clean and sanitize.

3. **Cookware Set:** Invest in a set of high-quality pots and pans, including a skillet, saucepan, and stockpot, to cover all your cooking needs.

4. **Blender or Food Processor:** These versatile appliances are perfect for making smoothies, sauces, and purees.

5. **Measuring Cups and Spoons:** Accurate measuring is crucial for following recipes and ensuring consistent results.

6. **Storage Containers:** Stock up on a variety of storage containers for storing leftovers, meal prep, and organizing pantry staples.

Pantry Essentials

Stocking your pantry with SIBO-friendly essentials will make meal planning and preparation much more straightforward. Here's a list of pantry staples to get you started:

- **Proteins**: Canned tuna, salmon, chicken, and turkey; frozen fish filets; eggs.
- **Vegetables**: Canned tomatoes, artichoke hearts, olives; frozen vegetables (e.g., spinach, broccoli,).
- **Fruits**: Fresh or frozen berries; canned fruits packed in water or juice (e.g., pineapple, peaches).
- **Grains and Seeds**: Quinoa, rice (white or brown), chia seeds, flaxseeds.
- **Nuts and Nut Butters:** Almonds, walnuts, cashews; almond butter, peanut butter (check for added sugars and oils).
- **Oils and Vinegars**: Olive oil, coconut oil, apple cider vinegar, balsamic vinegar.
- **Herbs and Spices:** Basil, oregano, thyme, rosemary, turmeric, ginger, cinnamon.

- **Condiments**: Coconut aminos, mustard, salsa, hot sauce (check for added sugars and artificial ingredients)

Shopping Tips

Navigating the grocery store can be overwhelming, especially when you're following a specific diet. Here are some tips to help you shop smart and make SIBO-friendly choices:

1. **Plan Ahead:** Take some time to plan your meals for the week and create a shopping list to avoid impulse purchases.
2. **Read Labels:** Always read food labels carefully to check for ingredients that may contain hidden FODMAPs or other potential triggers.
3. **Shop the organic produce:** Focus on shopping the area of the grocery store where you'll find

fresh produce, meats, and dairy alternatives.

4. **Buy in Bulk**: Consider buying non-perishable items like grains, seeds, and nuts in bulk to save money and reduce waste.

5. **Explore Specialty Stores**: Look for specialty stores or online retailers that offer a wide range of SIBO-friendly products and ingredients.

By equipping your kitchen with the right tools and stocking up on essential pantry items, you'll be well-prepared to embark on your SIBO diet journey. With these practical tips and resources, you'll find it easier than ever to create delicious, nourishing meals that support your gut health and overall well-being.

Chapter 4:

SIBO-Friendly Cooking Techniques.

Now that you have gotten your kitchen set up and pantry stocked with SIBO-friendly essentials, it's time to master some cooking techniques that will help you create delicious meals while adhering to the SIBO diet.

Sauteing, Steaming, and Roasting:

Understanding various cooking methods is essential for creating diverse and flavorful meals on the SIBO diet. Here's a breakdown of three versatile techniques you'll frequently use:

Sauteing: This quick and easy method involves cooking food in a pan with a small amount of oil or fat over medium-high heat. It's perfect for vegetables, proteins like chicken or fish, and even grains like quinoa or rice. Remember to keep an eye on your ingredients and stir frequently to prevent burning.

Steaming: Steaming is a gentle cooking method that preserves the natural flavors and nutrients of foods. Simply place your vegetables, fish, or poultry in a steamer basket over boiling water and cook until tender. Steaming is an excellent way to cook vegetables while keeping them crisp and vibrant.

Roasting: Roasting involves cooking food in an oven at a high temperature, allowing for caramelization and enhanced flavor. It's ideal for root vegetables, meats, and even some fruits. Preheat your oven, spread your ingredients on a baking sheet, drizzle with oil, and roast until golden and tender.

Flavoring Without FODMAPs:

Flavoring your dishes without FODMAPs doesn't mean sacrificing taste. Here are some SIBO-friendly ingredients and techniques to add depth and complexity to your meals:

Herbs and Spices: Fresh or dried herbs like basil, oregano, thyme, and rosemary can elevate your dishes' flavor without adding FODMAPs. Experiment with spices like turmeric, ginger, and cinnamon to add warmth and depth.

Citrus Zest and Juice: Lemon, lime, and orange zest and juice can brighten up your dishes and add a refreshing citrusy kick.

Infused Oils: Infuse olive or coconut oil with herbs, garlic, or chili flakes to create flavorful oils for cooking and dressing salads.

Homemade Sauces and Dressings: Make your own sauces and dressings using SIBO-friendly ingredients like coconut aminos, mustard, vinegar, and herbs.

Meal Prep Tips

Meal prep can be a game-changer when following the SIBO diet, saving you time and ensuring you have nourishing meals ready to go. Here are some tips to help you get started:

1. **Plan Your Meals:** Take some time each week to plan your meals, including breakfast, lunch, dinner, and snacks. This will help you create a balanced and varied diet.
2. **Batch Cooking:** Prepare large batches of staple ingredients like grains, proteins, and vegetables to mix and match throughout the week.

3. **Use Storage Containers:** Invest in a variety of storage containers to portion out meals and snacks, making it easy to grab and go.
4. **Label and Date:** Always label and date your meals and ingredients to keep track of what's in your fridge and when it was prepared.
5. **Freeze Extras:** If you have made more than you can eat, freeze leftovers in individual portions for easy meals on busy days.

By mastering these cooking techniques, flavoring strategies, and meal prep tips, you'll be well-equipped to create delicious and satisfying SIBO-friendly meals that support your gut health and overall well-being.

Chapter 5:

SIBO- Friendly Breakfasts Recipes

Breakfast is often considered the most important meal of the day, setting the tone for your energy levels and digestive comfort. In this chapter, we will ll explore a variety of SIBO-friendly breakfast options to kickstart your day, including low-FODMAP smoothies, grain-free pancakes, and egg-based dishes. We'll also provide dietary information and modifications for those with coexisting conditions to help you make these recipes to your individual needs.

1. Low-FODMAP Smoothies

Smoothies are a quick and convenient way to pack in nutrients while keeping your breakfast light and refreshing.

Here's a simple and delicious low-FODMAP smoothie recipe to start your day right:

Blueberry Banana Smoothie

Ingredients:
- 1/2 cup blueberries (fresh or frozen)
- 1/2 ripe banana
- 1 cup unsweetened almond milk
- 1 tbsp chia seeds (optional)
- 1 tbsp almond butter (optional)
- Ice cubes (optional)

Instructions:
1. Combine all ingredients in a blender.
2. Blend until smooth and creamy.
3. Pour into a glass and enjoy!

Nutritional Information (per serving):
Calories: 180
Protein: 4g
Carbohydrates: 28g

Fat: 7g
Fiber: 6g

Modifications:
In case of a coexisting disease like diabetes or need to watch your blood sugar levels, consider reducing the amount of banana or omitting it altogether. You can also add a sugar-free protein powder for added protein without the extra carbs.

2. Grain-Free Pancakes

Who says you can't enjoy pancakes on a SIBO diet? These grain-free pancakes are fluffy, flavorful, and perfect for a weekend brunch or special occasion.

Coconut Flour Pancakes

Ingredients:
- 1/4 cup coconut flour
- 2 eggs
- 1/2 cup unsweetened almond milk

- 1 tbsp coconut oil, melted
- 1/2 tsp baking powder
- 1/2 tsp vanilla extract
- Pinch of salt

Instructions:

1. In a bowl, whisk together eggs, almond milk, melted coconut oil, and vanilla extract.

2. Add coconut flour, baking powder, and salt. Mix until well combined.

3. Heat a non-stick skillet or griddle over medium heat.

4. Drop batter by spoonfuls onto the skillet and cook until bubbles form on the surface.

5. Flip and cook for another 1-2 minutes until golden brown.

6. Serve warm with your favorite toppings.

Nutritional Information (per serving, makes 2 pancakes):

- Calories: 180
- Protein: 8g

- Carbohydrates: 10g
- Fat: 12g
- Fiber: 5g

Modifications:
If you have a nut allergy, replace almond milk with another low-FODMAP milk alternative like lactose-free cow's milk or oat milk. You can also use ghee instead of coconut oil for a dairy-free option.

Egg-Based Dishes

Eggs are a versatile and nutritious option for breakfast, offering a good source of protein and essential nutrients. Here are two egg-based dishes to add variety to your morning routine:

Spinach and Feta Omelette

Ingredients:
- 2 eggs
- 1/4 cup spinach, chopped
- 2 tbsp feta cheese, crumbled

- Salt and pepper to taste
- 1 tsp olive oil or ghee

Instructions:
1. In a bowl, whisk eggs and season with salt and pepper.
2. Heat olive oil or ghee in a non-stick skillet over medium heat.
3. Add chopped spinach and sauté until wilted.
4. Pour whisked eggs over the spinach, tilting the pan to spread evenly.
5. Cook until the edges are set, then sprinkle feta cheese over one half of the omelette.
6. Fold the omelette in half and cook for another minute or until cheese is melted.
7. Slide onto a plate and enjoy!

Nutritional Information (per serving):
- **Calories**: 220
- **Protein**: 14g
- **Carbohydrates**: 2g

- **Fat**: 17g
- **Fiber**: 1g

Modifications:
If you have lactose intolerance or a dairy allergy, omit the feta cheese or replace it with a lactose-free or dairy-free cheese alternative. You can also add extra vegetables like bell peppers or tomatoes for added flavor and nutrients.

Spinach and Tomato Frittata

Ingredients:
- 6 large eggs
- 1 cup fresh spinach, chopped
- 1/2 cup cherry tomatoes, halved
- 1/4 cup dairy-free milk (almond milk or oat milk)
- 1/2 tsp: salt
- 1/4 tsp black pepper
- 1 tbsp olive oil

Instructions

1. Preheat your oven to 375°F (190°C).

2. Wash and chop the spinach. Halve the cherry tomatoes.

3. In a mixing bowl, whisk together the eggs, dairy-free milk, salt, and black pepper until well combined.

4. In an oven-safe skillet, heat olive oil over medium heat. Add the chopped spinach and cherry tomatoes to the skillet and sauté for 2-3 minutes until the spinach wilts and tomatoes soften.

5. Pour the whisked egg mixture over the sautéed vegetables in the skillet, ensuring an even distribution.

6. Cook the frittata on the stovetop for 3-4 minutes, or until the edges start to set.

7. Transfer the skillet to the preheated oven and bake for 10-12 minutes, or until the frittata is set and golden on top.

8. Remove from the oven and let it cool slightly. Slice the frittata into wedges and serve warm.

Nutritional Information (per serving):

- **Calories**: 120
- **Protein**: 9g
- **Carbohydrates**: 2g
- **Fat**: 8g
- **Fiber**: 1g

Modifications:

- **Dairy-Free**: This recipe is already dairy-free. However, you

can use regular milk if you don't
have lactose intolerance.

- **Low-FODMAP**: Cherry tomatoes
  and spinach are considered
  low-FODMAP in moderate
  servings. Adjust the portion sizes
  based on your tolerance levels.

By incorporating these SIBO-friendly
breakfast options into your morning
routine, you'll be setting yourself up for
a day of balanced energy and digestive
comfort. Feel free to experiment with
different ingredients and flavors to find
what works best for you.

Chapter 6:

Soups and Salads

Soups and salads are versatile dishes that can be both satisfying and nourishing, making them perfect additions to your SIBO-friendly meals.

1. Gut-Healing Bone Broth

Bone broth is a nutrient-rich liquid that can support gut health and digestion. It's packed with amino acids, collagen, and minerals that help repair and nourish the gut lining. Here's a simple bone broth recipe to try:

Basic Bone Broth

Ingredients:
- 2-3 lbs beef or chicken bones (preferably organic)
- 2 carrots, chopped

- 2 celery stalks, chopped
- 1 onion, quartered
- 3-4 cloves garlic, smashed
- 2 bay leaves
- 1 tbsp apple cider vinegar
- Water to cover

Instructions:
1. Place bones in a large stockpot and cover with water.
2. Add chopped vegetables, garlic, bay leaves, and apple cider vinegar.
3. Bring to a boil, then reduce heat to low and simmer for 12-24 hours, skimming off any foam that rises to the top.
4. Strain the broth through a fine-mesh sieve or cheesecloth and discard solids.
5. Let cool, then store in the refrigerator for up to 5 days or freeze for later use.

Nutritional Information (per cup):
- **Calories**: 40
- **Protein**: 6g
- **Carbohydrates**: 2g

- **Fat**: 1g
- **Fiber**: 0g

Modifications:

If you have histamine intolerance, consider simmering the bone broth for a shorter time (4-6 hours) to reduce histamine levels. You can also use a combination of chicken and fish bones for a lower histamine option.

2. Fresh and Flavorful Salads

Salads are a fantastic way to incorporate a variety of nutrient-dense ingredients into your diet. Here's a simple and refreshing salad recipe .

Greek Cucumber Salad

Ingredients:

- 2 cucumbers, diced
- 1 cup cherry tomatoes, halved
- 1/2 red onion, thinly sliced
- 1/4 cup Kalamata olives, pitted

- 1/4 cup feta cheese, crumbled (optional)
- 2 tbsp olive oil
- 1 tbsp red wine vinegar
- 1 tsp dried oregano
- Salt and pepper to taste

Instructions:

1. In a large bowl, combine diced cucumbers, cherry tomatoes, red onion, and Kalamata olives.

2. In a small bowl, whisk together olive oil, red wine vinegar, dried oregano, salt, and pepper.

3. Pour dressing over the salad and toss to combine.

4. Sprinkle crumbled feta cheese on top if using.

5. Serve chilled and enjoy!

Nutritional Information (per serving):*

- Calories: 120
- Protein: 2g
- Carbohydrates: 8g

- Fat: 9g
- Fiber: 2g

Modifications:
If you have a dairy allergy or lactose intolerance, omit the feta cheese or replace it with a dairy-free cheese alternative. You can also add grilled chicken or tofu for added protein.

Creamy Vegetable Soups

Creamy vegetable soups are comforting and nourishing, making them a perfect choice for chilly days or when you're craving something warm and satisfying. Here's a delicious and creamy vegetable soup recipe to try:

Butternut Squash Soup

Ingredients:
- 1 medium butternut squash, peeled, seeded, and cubed
- 1 carrot, chopped

- 1 celery stalk, chopped
- 4 cups vegetable broth
- 1 cup coconut milk
- 2 tbsp olive oil or ghee
- 1 tsp dried thyme
- Salt and pepper to taste

Instructions:

1. In a large pot, heat olive oil or ghee over medium heat.

2. Add carrot, celery and Sauté until softened.

3. Add cubed butternut squash, dried thyme, salt, and pepper. Cook for a few minutes.

4. Pour in vegetable broth and bring to a boil. Reduce heat and simmer until squash is tender.

5. Use an immersion blender or transfer to a blender to puree until smooth.

6. Stir in coconut milk and heat through.

7. Adjust seasoning if needed and serve hot.

Nutritional Information (per serving):

- Calories: 200
- Protein: 3g
- Carbohydrates: 25g
- Fat: 12g
- Fiber: 5g

Modifications:

If you have a coconut allergy or intolerance, replace coconut milk with lactose-free cow's milk, almond milk, or oat milk. You can also add a dollop of lactose-free sour cream or yogurt for added creaminess.

Chapter 7:

Meat and Poultry Dishes

Meat and poultry dishes can be hearty, satisfying, and packed with essential nutrients. Let's look at Some of them.

1. Herb-Roasted Chicken

Roasting a whole chicken with herbs infuses it with flavor while keeping it moist and tender. This dish is perfect for a Sunday dinner or special occasion.

Ingredients:
- 1 whole chicken (about 3-4 lbs), giblets removed
- 2 tbsp olive oil
- 2 cloves gar
- 1 tsp dried rosemary
- 1 tsp dried thyme
- 1 tsp dried oregano
- Salt and pepper to taste

Instructions:

1. Preheat the oven to 425°F (220°C).

2. In a small bowl, combine olive oil, dried rosemary, thyme, oregano, salt, and pepper to make a herb rub.

3. Pat the chicken dry with paper towels and rub the herb mixture all over the chicken, including under the skin.

4. Place the chicken in a roasting pan breast side up.

5. Roast for about 60-75 minutes, or until the internal temperature reaches 165°F (75°C) when tested with a meat thermometer.

6. Let the chicken rest for 10 minutes before carving.

7. Serve hot with your favorite sides.

Nutritional Information (per serving):

- Calories: 300
- Protein: 30g
- Carbohydrates: 0g
- Fat: 20g

- Fiber: 0g

Modifications:
If you have high cholesterol or cardiovascular issues, consider removing the skin before eating to reduce the fat content. You can also use skinless chicken breasts or thighs for a leaner option.

2. Beef Stir-Fry with Veggies

Ingredients:
- 1 lb beef sirloin or flank steak, thinly sliced
- 2 cups mixed vegetables (bell peppers, broccoli, carrots, snap peas)
- 2 cloves garlic, minced
- 2 tbsp soy sauce or tamari (low-sodium)
- 1 tbsp olive oil or sesame oil
- 1 tsp ginger, grated (if tolerated)
- Salt and pepper to taste

Instructions:

1. In a large skillet or wok, heat olive oil or sesame oil over medium-high heat.

2. Add minced garlic and grated ginger, sauté for 1 minute.

3. Add sliced beef and stir-fry until browned, about 3-4 minutes.

4. Add mixed vegetables and continue to stir-fry until tender-crisp, about 5-6 minutes.

5. Stir in soy sauce or tamari, and season with salt and pepper to taste.

6. Cook for another 1-2 minutes, stirring continuously.

7. Remove from heat and serve hot.

Nutritional Information (per serving):

- Calories: 250
- Protein: 25g
- Carbohydrates: 10g
- Fat: 12g
- Fiber: 3g

***Modifications**:*

If you have gluten sensitivity or intolerance, use gluten-free tamari instead of soy sauce. You can also add more vegetables and reduce the amount of meat to lower the fat content.

3. Lamb Kebabs with Mint Sauce

Lamb kebabs are nutritious and delicious, especially when paired with a refreshing mint sauce. This dish is perfect for grilling season or a weekend barbecue.

Ingredients:
- 1 lb lamb loin or leg, cubed
- 1 bell pepper, cut into chunks
- 1 red onion, cut into chunks
- 2 cloves garlic, minced
- 2 tbsp olive oil
- 1 tsp dried rosemary
- Salt and pepper to taste

Mint Sauce:

- 1/2 cup fresh mint leaves, finely chopped
- 1/4 cup plain yogurt or coconut yogurt (for dairy-free)
- 1 tbsp lemon juice
- Salt to taste

Instructions:

1. In a bowl, combine cubed lamb, olive oil, minced garlic, dried rosemary, salt, and pepper. Marinate for at least 30 minutes.

2. Thread marinated lamb, bell pepper, and red onion onto skewers.

3. Preheat grill or grill pan over medium-high heat.

4. Grill kebabs for 10-12 minutes, turning occasionally, until lamb is cooked to your liking.

5. While the kebabs are grilling, prepare the mint sauce by combining chopped mint leaves, yogurt, lemon juice, and salt in a bowl. Mix well.

6. Serve hot kebabs with mint sauce on the side.

Nutritional Information (per serving, includes mint sauce):
- Calories: 320
- Protein: 30g
- Carbohydrates: 8g
- Fat: 18g
- Fiber: 2g

Modifications:
If you have lactose intolerance or a dairy allergy, use coconut yogurt instead of dairy-based yogurt for the mint sauce. You can also add more vegetables like zucchini or cherry tomatoes to the kebabs to increase fiber and reduce the meat portion size.

Chapter 8:

Fish and Seafood Recipes

1. Lemon Herb Grilled Fish:

Grilled fish is a simple yet delicious dish that's perfect for a light and healthy meal. The combination of fresh herbs and zesty lemon adds a burst of flavor to the fish.

Ingredients:
- 4 fish filets (such as salmon, trout, or cod)
- 2 tbsp olive oil
- 2 cloves garlic, minced
- 1 tbsp fresh parsley, chopped
- 1 tbsp fresh dill, chopped
- Zest and juice of 1 lemon
- Salt and pepper to taste

Instructions:

1. Preheat grill or grill pan over medium-high heat.

2. In a bowl, combine olive oil, minced garlic, chopped parsley, dill, lemon zest, lemon juice, salt, and pepper to make a marinade.

3. Pat the fish fillets dry with paper towels and coat them with the marinade.

4. Grill fish for 3-4 minutes per side, or until opaque and easily flaked with a fork.

5. Remove from grill and serve hot with your favorite sides.

Nutritional Information (per serving):
- Calories: 250
- Protein: 30g
- Carbohydrates: 2g
- Fat: 14g
- Fiber: 0g

Modifications:
If you have high cholesterol or cardiovascular issues, opt for lean fish

like cod or tilapia. You can also reduce the amount of olive oil in the marinade to lower the fat content.

2. Shrimp and Vegetable Skewers

Shrimp and vegetable skewers are a fun and colorful way to enjoy seafood. Grilling adds a smoky flavor to the shrimp and veggies, making this dish irresistible.

Ingredients:
- 1 lb large shrimp, peeled and deveined
- 2 bell peppers, cut into chunks
- 1 zucchini, sliced
- 2 tbsp olive oil
- 2 cloves garlic, minced (optional, if not tolerated)
- 1 tsp paprika
- Salt and pepper to taste

Instructions:

1. Preheat grill or grill pan over medium-high heat.

2. In a bowl, combine olive oil, minced garlic, paprika, salt, and pepper to make a marinade.

3. Thread shrimp and vegetables onto skewers, alternating between shrimp, bell peppers, red onion, and zucchini.

4. Brush skewers with the marinade.

5. Grill skewers for 2-3 minutes per side, or until shrimp are pink and vegetables are tender.

6. Serve hot with a squeeze of fresh lemon juice.

Nutritional Information (per serving):

- Calories: 200
- Protein: 25g
- Carbohydrates: 8g
- Fat: 8g
- Fiber: 2g
-

Modifications:

If you have histamine intolerance, consider using fresh shrimp instead of frozen to reduce histamine levels. You can also skip the garlic and paprika in the marinade and use olive oil with lemon juice for a simpler flavor profile.

3. Coconut Curry Seafood Stew

This coconut curry seafood stew is a comforting and aromatic dish that's perfect for cooler days. The combination of seafood, coconut milk, and spices creates a nutrient dense meal.

Ingredients:
- 1 lb mixed seafood (such as shrimp, scallops, and fish filets)
- 1 can (13.5 oz) coconut milk
- 1 bell pepper, diced
- 1 onion, diced
- 1/2 clove garlic, minced (optional)
- 1 tbsp curry powder
- 1 tsp turmeric
- 1 tsp ginger, grated (optional)

- 2 tbsp olive oil
- Salt and pepper to taste
- Fresh cilantro for garnish

Instructions:
1. In a large pot, heat olive oil over medium heat.
2. Add diced onion, bell pepper, and minced garlic. Sauté until softened.
3. Stir in curry powder, turmeric, and grated ginger. Cook for another minute.
4. Add coconut milk and bring to a simmer.
5. Add mixed seafood and cook for 5-7 minutes, or until seafood is cooked through.
6. Season with salt and pepper to taste.
7. Garnish with fresh cilantro before serving.

Nutritional Information (per serving):
- Calories: 320
- Protein: 20g
- Carbohydrates: 10g

- Fat: 24g
- Fiber: 2g

Modifications:

If you have a nut allergy, use another type of milk (such as lactose-free cow's milk or oat milk) instead of coconut milk. You can also adjust the amount of curry powder and spices to suit your taste preferences.

Chapter 9:

Vegetable-Packed Mains

Vegetables are a fantastic way to add color, nutrients, and texture to your meals while providing essential vitamins and minerals. Whether you're following a vegetarian lifestyle or looking to incorporate more veggies into your diet, these recipes are sure to please your taste.

1. Zucchini Noodles with Pesto

Zucchini noodles, also known as "zoodles," are a fantastic low-carb alternative to traditional pasta. Paired with homemade pesto, this dish is light, flavorful, and satisfying.

Ingredients:
- 4 medium zucchinis, spiralized
- 1 cup fresh basil leaves

- 1/4 cup pine nuts or walnuts
- 2 cloves garlic (if tolerated)
- 1/4 cup olive oil
- 1/4 cup grated Parmesan cheese (optional)
- Salt and pepper to taste

Instructions:

1. In a food processor, combine basil leaves, pine nuts, garlic, olive oil, and Parmesan cheese (if using). Blend until smooth.

2. In a large skillet, heat a drizzle of olive oil over medium heat.

3. Add zucchini noodles and sauté for 3-4 minutes, or until tender but still slightly crunchy.

4. Toss zucchini noodles with pesto until well coated.

5. Season with salt and pepper to taste.

6. Serve hot, garnished with extra Parmesan cheese and pine nuts if desired.

Nutritional Information (per serving):

- Calories: 200
- Protein: 4g
- Carbohydrates: 8g
- Fat: 18g
- Fiber: 3g

Modifications:

If you have a nut allergy, omit the pine nuts or walnuts and use seeds like sunflower or pumpkin seeds instead.

For a dairy-free option, skip the Parmesan cheese or use a dairy-free alternative.

2. Stuffed Bell Peppers

Stuffed bell peppers are a versatile and colorful dish that's perfect for lunch or dinner. You can customize the filling based on your preferences and dietary needs.

Ingredients:

- 4 large bell peppers, tops removed and seeds removed
- 1 lb ground turkey or chicken
- 1 onion, diced
- 1/2 clove garlic, minced (optional)
- 1 zucchini, diced
- 1 cup cooked quinoa or cauliflower rice
- 1 cup tomato sauce
- 1 tsp dried herbs (such as oregano, basil, or thyme)
- Salt and pepper to taste
- Olive oil for cooking

Instructions:

1. Preheat the oven to 375°F (190°C).

2. In a large skillet, heat olive oil over medium heat.

3. Add diced onion, minced garlic, and diced zucchini. Sauté until softened.

4. Add ground turkey or chicken, breaking it apart with a spoon, and cook until browned.

5. Stir in cooked quinoa or cauliflower rice, tomato sauce, dried herbs, salt, and pepper.

6. Spoon the filling into the hollowed-out bell peppers.

7. Place stuffed bell peppers in a baking dish and cover with foil.

8. Bake for 30-35 minutes, or until peppers are tender.

9. Serve hot with a side salad or additional tomato sauce if desired.

Nutritional Information (per serving):

- Calories: 300
- Protein: 25g
- Carbohydrates: 20g
- Fat: 12g
- Fiber: 5g

Modifications:

If you have a grain sensitivity or allergy, omit the quinoa and use additional vegetables or a grain-free alternative like cauliflower rice. For a vegetarian option, use plant-based ground meat or lentils instead of turkey or chicken.

Chapter 10:

Quick and Easy Sides

Side dishes are great part of any meal, adding flavor, color, and nutritional value to your plate. Let's take a look at some quick and easy side dishes that are perfect for complementing your main courses.

1. Ginger Roasted Brussels Sprouts.

Roasting Brussels sprouts brings out their natural sweetness and adds a good caramelized flavor. Ginger and olive oil lifts this simple side dish to new heights.

Ingredients:
- 1 lb Brussels sprouts, trimmed and halved
- 2 tbsp olive oil
- 1 finger of ginger, minced

- Salt and pepper to taste

Instructions:

1. Preheat oven to 400°F (200°C).

2. In a large bowl, toss Brussels sprouts with olive oil, minced ginger, salt, and pepper until well coated.

3. Spread Brussels sprouts in a single layer on a baking sheet.

4. Roast for 20-25 minutes, or until Brussels sprouts are tender and golden brown, stirring halfway through.

5. Serve hot as a side to your favorite main course.

Nutritional Information (per serving):

- Calories: 100
- Protein: 4g
- Carbohydrates: 10g
- Fat: 7g
- Fiber: 4g

Modifications:

If you have a ginger intolerance, omit the garlic or use ginger-infused olive oil. For a nuttier flavor, sprinkle roasted Brussels sprouts with chopped almonds or pecans before serving.

2. Mashed Root Vegetables

Mashed root vegetables are a comforting and nutritious side dish that pairs well with a variety of main courses. You can mix your favorite root vegetables to create a colorful and delicious side for your meal.

Ingredients:
- 2 cups mixed root vegetables (such as carrots, parsnips, and sweet potatoes), peeled and diced
- 2 tbsp olive oil or ghee
- 1/4 cup unsweetened almond milk or lactose-free milk
- Salt and pepper to taste

Instructions:

1. In a large pot, bring water to a boil and add diced root vegetables.

2. Cook until vegetables are tender, about 15-20 minutes.

3. Drain cooked vegetables and transfer to a large mixing bowl.

4. Add olive oil or ghee and almond milk.

5. Mash vegetables using a potato masher or fork until desired consistency is reached.

6. Season with salt and pepper to taste.

7. Serve hot alongside your favorite protein.

Nutritional Information (per serving):

- Calories: 150
- Protein: 2g
- Carbohydrates: 20g
- Fat: 7g
- Fiber: 4g

Modifications:

If you have a nut allergy, use lactose-free cow's milk or oat milk instead of almond milk. You can also add fresh herbs like rosemary or thyme for extra flavor.

3. Steamed Asparagus with Lemon Butter

Steamed asparagus with lemon butter is a simple yet elegant side dish that's perfect for any occasion. The sweet aroma of lemon and butter complement the tender asparagus beautifully.

Ingredients:
- 1 lb asparagus spears, trimmed
- 2 tbsp unsalted butter or dairy-free alternative
- Zest and juice of 1 lemon
- Salt and pepper to taste

Instructions:
1. Fill a large pot with a few inches of water and bring to a boil.

2. Place asparagus spears in a steamer basket and set over the boiling water.
3. Cover and steam for 3-5 minutes, or until asparagus is tender but still crisp.
4. While asparagus is steaming, melt butter in a small saucepan over low heat.
5. Stir in lemon zest and juice, and season with salt and pepper.
6. Drizzle lemon butter over steamed asparagus just before serving.

Nutritional Information (per serving):

- Calories: 80
- Protein: 3g
- Carbohydrates: 5g
- Fat: 7g
- Fiber: 2g

Modifications:

If you have a dairy intolerance, use a dairy-free butter alternative. You can also add minced garlic or a pinch of red pepper flakes to the lemon butter for an extra kick of flavor.

Chapter 11:

Recipe for Snacks and Appetizers

1. Spiced Nuts

Spiced nuts are a crunchy and tasty snack that's perfect for munching on the go or serving to guests. The combination of sweet, salty, and spicy flavors makes these nuts irresistible.

Ingredients:
- 2 cups mixed nuts (such as almonds, walnuts, and pecans)
- 1 tbsp olive oil
- 1 tbsp maple syrup
- 1 tsp ground cumin
- 1/2 tsp smoked paprika
- 1/4 tsp cayenne pepper (optional)
- Salt to taste

Instructions:

1. Preheat the oven to 350°F (175°C).

2. In a large bowl, combine mixed nuts, olive oil, maple syrup, ground cumin, smoked paprika, cayenne pepper (if using), and salt. Toss until nuts are evenly coated.

3. Spread nut mixture in a single layer on a baking sheet lined with parchment paper.

4. Bake for 10-12 minutes, stirring halfway through, or until nuts are golden and fragrant.

5. Remove from the oven and let cool completely before serving or storing in an airtight container.

Nutritional Information (per serving):

- Calories: 200
- Protein: 5g
- Carbohydrates: 8g
- Fat: 18g
- Fiber: 3g

Modifications:

If you have a nut allergy, you can use seeds like pumpkin or sunflower seeds as a substitute. For a sweeter version, increase the amount of maple syrup

2. Veggie Sticks with Hummus

Veggie sticks with hummus are a classic and nutritious snack that's perfect for satisfying your mid-day cravings. The combination of crunchy veggies and creamy hummus provides a great satisfaction

Ingredients:
- 2 carrots, peeled and cut into sticks
- 2 celery stalks, cut into sticks
- 1 bell pepper, sliced
- 1 cup cherry tomatoes, halved
- 1 cup hummus (store-bought or homemade)

Instructions:

1. Wash and prepare all vegetables as directed.

2. Arrange veggie sticks and cherry tomatoes on a serving platter.

3. Place hummus in a small bowl in the center of the platter.

4. Serve immediately and enjoy!

Nutritional Information (per serving):
- Calories: 150
- Protein: 6g
- Carbohydrates: 20g
- Fat: 6g
- Fiber: 8g

Modifications:

If you have a legume intolerance, consider making a bean-free hummus using roasted cauliflower or zucchini. You can also use cucumber slices or broccoli florets as additional veggie options.

3. Olive Tapenade

Olive tapenade is a nutritious spread made from olives, capers, and herbs. It's perfect for serving as an appetizer with crackers or sliced veggies, or as a topping for grilled meats and fish.

Ingredients:
- 1 cup pitted Kalamata olives
- 2 tbsp capers, rinsed and drained
- 2 cloves garlic
- 1/4 cup fresh parsley leaves
- 2 tbsp olive oil
- 1 tbsp lemon juice
- Salt and pepper to taste

Instructions:
1. In a food processor, combine Kalamata olives, capers, garlic, and parsley.
2. Pulse until mixture is coarsely chopped.
3. With the food processor running, drizzle in olive oil and lemon juice until combined.

4. Season with salt and pepper to taste.

5. Transfer olive tapenade to a serving bowl and refrigerate for at least 30 minutes to allow flavors to meld.

6. Serve with crackers, sliced baguette, or veggie sticks.

Nutritional Information (per serving):
- Calories: 80
- Protein: 1g
- Carbohydrates: 4g
- Fat: 7g
- Fiber: 2g

Modifications:

If you have a garlic intolerance, omit the garlic or use garlic-infused olive oil. You can also add fresh herbs like basil or thyme for an extra layer of flavor.

Chapter 12:

Recipes for Desserts

Who said you have to skip dessert while following a special diet? In this chapter, we will try some decadent desserts that are not only delicious but also friendly to those following the SIBO diet.

1. Chocolate Avocado Pudding.

Creamy, rich, and chocolatey – this avocado pudding is a guilt-free dessert that's sure to satisfy your chocolate cravings. Avocado adds creaminess while also providing healthy fats and nutrients.

Ingredients:
- 2 ripe avocados, peeled and pitted
- 1/4 cup unsweetened cocoa powder
- 1/4 cup maple syrup

- 1/4 cup unsweetened almond milk or lactose-free milk
- 1 tsp vanilla extract
- Pinch of salt

Instructions:

1. In a food processor or blender, combine avocados, cocoa powder, maple syrup, almond milk, vanilla extract, and salt.

2. Blend until smooth and creamy, scraping down the sides as needed.

3. Taste and adjust sweetness if needed by adding more maple syrup or honey.

4. Transfer pudding to serving dishes and refrigerate for at least 30 minutes before serving.

5. Garnish with fresh berries or shaved chocolate, if desired.

Nutritional Information (per serving):

- Calories: 200
- Protein: 3g
- Carbohydrates: 20g

- Fat: 14g
- Fiber: 7g

Modifications:

If you have a nut allergy, use coconut milk or oat milk instead of almond milk. For a sweeter pudding, add more maple syrup to taste.

2. Coconut Macaroons

These coconut macaroons are sweet, chewy, and packed with coconut flavor. They're also gluten-free and dairy-free, making them a perfect dessert option for those with dietary restrictions.

Ingredients:

- 2 cups unsweetened shredded coconut
- 1/2 cup maple syrup or
- 2 egg whites
- 1 tsp vanilla extract
- Pinch of salt

Instructions:

1. Preheat the oven to 325°F (160°C). Line a baking sheet with parchment paper.

2. In a large bowl, combine shredded coconut, maple syrup, vanilla extract, and salt.

3. In a separate bowl, beat egg whites until stiff peaks form.

4. Gently fold beaten egg whites into the coconut mixture until well combined.

5. Drop spoonfuls of the mixture onto the prepared baking sheet, forming small mounds.

6. Bake for 20-25 minutes, or until macaroons are golden brown.

7. Let cool completely before serving.

Nutritional Information (per serving, about 2 macaroons):
- Calories: 120
- Protein: 2g
- Carbohydrates: 15g
- Fat: 6g
- Fiber: 2g

Modifications:

If you have an egg allergy, you can try using aquafaba (the liquid from canned chickpeas) as a substitute. For a sweeter version, drizzle melted dark chocolate over the cooled macaroons.

3. Berry Parfait with Coconut Cream.

This berry parfait with coconut cream is a refreshing and delicious dessert that's perfect for showcasing fresh seasonal berries. The creamy coconut layer adds richness and a tropical twist.

Ingredients:

- 1 cup mixed berries (such as strawberries, blueberries, and raspberries)
- 1 can (14 oz) full-fat coconut milk, refrigerated overnight
- 2 tbsp maple syrup
- 1 tsp vanilla extract

Instructions:
1. Chill a mixing bowl in the freezer for 10 minutes.
2. Open the refrigerated can of coconut milk and scoop out the solid coconut cream that has risen to the top, leaving behind the liquid.
3. Place the solid coconut cream in the chilled mixing bowl.
4. Add maple syrup and vanilla extract to the coconut cream.
5. Beat with an electric mixer until light and fluffy, about 2-3 minutes.
6. Layer the coconut cream and mixed berries in serving glasses or bowls, starting with a layer of coconut cream followed by a layer of berries.
7. Repeat layers until all ingredients are used, ending with a layer of berries on top.
8. Refrigerate parfait for at least 30 minutes before

Chapter 13:

SIBO- Friendly Beverages and Smoothies

When it comes to maintaining good digestive health, what you drink is just as important as what you eat. In this chapter, we'll explore a variety of beverages and smoothies designed to support digestion, boost gut health, and also deliver a great taste.

1. Herbal Teas for Digestion

Herbal teas have been used for centuries to soothe digestive discomfort and promote overall well-being. Whether you're dealing with bloating, gas, or other digestive issues, these herbal teas can offer relief and comfort.

Ingredients:

- 1-2 tsp dried chamomile flowers or peppermint leaves
- 1 cup boiling water

Instructions:
1. Place dried chamomile flowers or peppermint leaves in a teapot or mug.
2. Pour boiling water over the herbs.
3. Cover and steep for 5-10 minutes.
4. Strain and enjoy warm.

Nutritional Information (per serving):
- Calories: 0
- Protein: 0g
- Carbohydrates: 0g
- Fat: 0g
- Fiber: 0g

Modifications:
If you have an allergy to chamomile or peppermint, try ginger tea or fennel tea instead. Always consult with a healthcare provider before trying new

herbal remedies, especially if you have underlying health conditions.

2. Gut-Healing Smoothies

Smoothies are a fantastic way to pack in nutrients while enjoying a delicious and refreshing drink. These gut-healing smoothies are loaded with ingredients that support digestive health, including fiber-rich fruits, probiotics, and anti-inflammatory ingredients.

Ingredients:
- 1 cup mixed berries (such as blueberries, strawberries, and raspberries)
- 1 ripe banana
- 1 cup unsweetened almond milk or lactose-free milk
- 1/2 cup plain Greek yogurt or dairy-free yogurt
- 1 tbsp chia seeds or ground flaxseeds
- 1 tsp maple syrup (optional)

Instructions:

1. Combine all ingredients in a blender.

2. Blend until smooth and creamy.

3. Taste and adjust sweetness if needed by adding maple syrup.

4. Pour into a glass and enjoy immediately.

Nutritional Information (per serving):

- Calories: 250
- Protein: 10g
- Carbohydrates: 40g
- Fat: 6g
- Fiber: 8g

Modifications:

If you have a nut allergy, use coconut milk or oat milk instead of almond milk.

For a dairy-free option, use dairy-free yogurt made from coconut milk or almonds.

3. Infused Water Recipes

Staying hydrated is crucial for overall health and digestion. Infusing water with fruits, herbs, and spices adds flavor without added sugars or artificial ingredients. These infused water recipes are refreshing, hydrating, and perfect for sipping throughout the day.

Ingredients:

A. Citrus Mint Infused Water:
- 1 lemon, sliced
- 1 lime, sliced
- a handful of fresh mint leaves
- 1 quart water

B. Cucumber Ginger Infused Water:
- 1/2 cucumber, sliced
- 1-inch piece of ginger, sliced
- 1 quart water

Instructions:

1. For each infused water recipe, combine the ingredients in a pitcher.

2. Fill the pitcher with water.

3. Refrigerate for at least 2 hours, or overnight, to allow flavors to infuse.

4. Serve chilled, with or without ice.

Nutritional Information (per serving):

- Calories: 0
- Protein: 0g
- Carbohydrates: 0g
- Fat: 0g
- Fiber: 0g

Modifications:

Feel free to experiment with different fruits, herbs, and spices based on your preferences and dietary restrictions. Always use fresh, organic ingredients when possible.

Chapter 14:

Fermented Foods for Gut Health:

Fermented foods are loaded with a lot of beneficial bacteria that can help support and balance your gut microbiome. Incorporating fermented foods into your diet is an excellent way to boost digestive health, improve nutrient absorption, and strengthen your immune system. Here, you will be guided through the process of making your own fermented foods at home.

1. DIY Sauerkraut

Sauerkraut is a classic fermented food made from cabbage that's rich in probiotics, vitamins, and minerals. Making your own sauerkraut at home is surprisingly simple and allows you to customize the flavors to your liking.

Ingredients:
- 1 head green cabbage, thinly sliced
- 1-2 tbsp sea salt
- **Optional**: caraway seeds, juniper berries, or other spices

Instructions:
1. In a large mixing bowl, combine sliced cabbage and salt.
2. Massage the cabbage with your hands for 5-10 minutes until it starts to release its juices.
3. Add optional spices if desired and mix well.
4. Pack the cabbage mixture tightly into a clean glass jar, pressing down to submerge the cabbage in its own juices.
5. Cover the jar with a lid, but don't seal it completely; gases produced during fermentation need to escape.
6. Store the jar at room temperature, away from direct sunlight, for 1-2 weeks.
7. Check the sauerkraut daily, pressing down on the cabbage to ensure it remains submerged.

8. Taste the sauerkraut after 1 week. If it's tangy enough for your liking, transfer the jar to the refrigerator to slow down the fermentation process.

Nutritional Information (per serving):

- Calories: 5
- Protein: 0g
- Carbohydrates: 1g
- Fat: 0g
- Fiber: 1g

Modifications:

If you have a sensitivity to cabbage or are following a low-FODMAP diet, you can use green cabbage sparingly or opt for other vegetables like carrots or cucumbers to make fermented foods.

2. Coconut Yogurt

Coconut yogurt is a dairy-free alternative to traditional yogurt that's rich, creamy, and packed with probiotics. Making coconut yogurt at home allows you to control the ingredients and avoid added sugars and preservatives.

Ingredients:

- 2 cans (14 oz each) full-fat coconut milk
- 2-3 probiotic capsules or 1/4 cup store-bought coconut yogurt with live cultures

Instructions:

1. Sterilize a glass jar and its lid by boiling them in water for 10 minutes or running them through a hot dishwasher cycle.
2. In a mixing bowl, whisk together the coconut milk and probiotic capsules or store-bought yogurt until well combined.
3. Pour the mixture into the sterilized glass jar.

4. Cover the jar with a clean cloth and secure it with a rubber band or string.

5. Place the jar in a warm spot, like a turned-off oven with the light on or a warm corner of your kitchen.

6. Let the yogurt ferment for 24-48 hours, checking periodically for desired tartness.

7. Once fermented, stir the yogurt, transfer it to the refrigerator, and chill for at least 4 hours before serving.

Nutritional Information (per serving):

- Calories: 150
- Protein: 2g
- Carbohydrates: 5g
- Fat: 14g
- Fiber: 1g

Modifications:

If you have a nut allergy, coconut yogurt may not be suitable. You can try making yogurt from dairy-free alternatives like almond milk or oat milk, following a similar fermentation process.

3. Fermented Pickles

Pickles are a popular fermented food that's crunchy, tangy, and perfect for snacking or adding to sandwiches and salads. Making your own fermented pickles allows you to skip the preservatives and enjoy the probiotic benefits.

Ingredients:
- 4-6 pickling cucumbers, washed and sliced into spears or rounds
- 2 cups water
- 1 tbsp sea salt
- **Optional**: garlic cloves, dill sprigs, peppercorns

Instructions:
1. In a large mixing bowl, dissolve sea salt in water to create a brine.

2. Place cucumber slices, along with any optional ingredients, into a clean glass jar.

3. Pour the brine over the cucumbers, ensuring they are completely submerged.

4. Place a weight on top of the cucumbers to keep them submerged under the brine.

5. Cover the jar with a lid, but leave it slightly loose to allow gasses to escape during fermentation.

6. Store the jar at room temperature, away from direct sunlight, for 1-2 weeks.

7. Check the pickles daily, skimming off any scum that forms on the surface.

8. Taste the pickles after 1 week. If they're tangy enough for your liking, transfer the jar to the refrigerator to slow down the fermentation process.

Nutritional Information (per serving):

- Calories: 5
- Protein: 0g

- Carbohydrates: 1g
- Fat: 0g
- Fiber: 0g

Modifications:

If you have a sensitivity to cucumbers or are following a low-FODMAP diet, you can experiment with other vegetables like carrots or green beans to make fermented pickles.

Chapter 15:

Meal Planning and Prepping.

Meal planning and prepping are very essential for success when following a specific diet like the SIBO diet. Planning your meals ahead of time not only saves you from last-minute stress but also ensures you have nutritious and gut-friendly options readily available.

Weekly Meal Plans:

Creating a weekly meal plan is a game-changer when it comes to sticking to a diet and saving time throughout the week. Here's a sample 7-day meal plan to inspire you:

Day 1:
Breakfast: Low-FODMAP smoothie with blueberries, spinach, and almond milk.

Lunch: Herb-roasted chicken with zucchini noodles.
Dinner: Coconut curry seafood stew.

Day 2:
Breakfast: Grain-free pancakes with maple syrup.

Lunch: Gut-healing bone broth soup.

Dinner: Beef stir-fry with veggies.

Day 3:
Breakfast: Egg scramble with spinach, tomatoes, and avocado.

Lunch: Stuffed bell peppers with ground turkey.

Dinner: Lemon herb grilled fish with steamed asparagus.

Day 4:

Breakfast: Chia seed pudding with mixed berries.

Lunch: Cauliflower fried rice with shrimp.

Dinner: Lamb kebabs with mint sauce and salad.

Day 5:
Breakfast: Coconut yogurt parfait with granola.

Lunch: Creamy vegetable soup.

Dinner: Chicken curry with cauliflower rice

Day 6:
Breakfast: Smoothie bowl with banana, berries, and coconut flakes.

Lunch: Zucchini noodles with pesto and grilled chicken.

Dinner: Beef and vegetable stew

Day 7:
Breakfast: Grain-free granola with almond milk.

Lunch: Salad with mixed greens, cherry tomatoes, cucumber, and grilled shrimp.

Dinner: Turkey meatballs with spaghetti squash.

Feel free to mix and match these recipes to suit your preferences and dietary needs. Planning your meals in advance allows you to create a shopping list, save money by buying in bulk, and reduce food waste.

Batch Cooking Tips

Batch cooking is a helpful time-saving strategy that involves preparing multiple meals at once to enjoy throughout the week. Here are some tips to get you started:

1. **Choose Versatile Ingredients:** Opt for ingredients that can be used in multiple dishes, such as roasted vegetables, grilled chicken, or cooked grains.

2. **Invest in Quality Containers**: Use airtight containers or meal prep containers to store your batch-cooked meals safely in the refrigerator or freezer.

3. **Label and Date**: Always label your containers with the meal name and date of preparation to keep track of freshness.

4. **Portion Control:** Divide your batch-cooked meals into individual portions to grab and go for easy lunches or dinners.

5. **Rotate Recipes**: To avoid meal fatigue, rotate between different recipes throughout the week, so you don't get bored with your meals.

Storage and Reheating Guidelines:

Proper storage and reheating can make a significant difference in preserving the flavor and texture of your prepared meals. Here are some guidelines to follow:

- **Refrigeration**: Store cooked meals in airtight containers in the refrigerator for up to 4 days.
- **Freezing**: For longer storage, freeze meals in freezer-safe containers for up to 3 months.
- **Reheating**: Reheat refrigerated or frozen meals in the microwave or oven until heated through. Stirring halfway through can help distribute heat evenly.

- **Safety First:** Always ensure that reheated meals reach an internal temperature of 165°F (74°C) to kill any bacteria.

Chapter 16:

Adapting Recipes for Special Diets:

Adapting recipes to meet specific dietary needs is a crucial skill that can make all the difference in enjoying a diverse and satisfying diet. Whether you're vegan, vegetarian, gluten-free, or dairy-free, there are plenty of delicious and nutritious options available to you.

Let's discuss ways to adapt recipes to accommodate these special diets without compromising on flavor or nutritional value.

Vegan and Vegetarian Options:

Adding more plant-based meals to your diet can be both delicious and beneficial for your health. Here's how you can adapt some of our recipes to be vegan or vegetarian-friendly:

1. Herb-Roasted Chicken → Herb-Roasted Tofu:

- Replace chicken with firm tofu slices.
- Use the same herb mixture for seasoning.
- Bake until tofu is golden and crispy.

2. Beef Stir-Fry with Veggies → Veggie Stir-Fry:

- Skip the beef and add extra veggies like bell peppers, broccoli, and snap peas.
- Use tamari or coconut aminos instead of soy sauce for a gluten-free option.

3. Lemon Herb Grilled Fish → Grilled Portobello Mushrooms:

- Substitute fish with large portobello mushroom caps.
- Marinate in lemon juice, olive oil, and herbs before grilling.

Gluten-Free Alternatives:

For those following a gluten-free diet, there are plenty of ways to enjoy your favorite dishes without gluten-containing ingredients:

1. Grain-Free Pancakes → Almond Flour Pancakes:

- Replace all-purpose flour with almond flour.
- Use a gluten-free baking powder if needed.

2. **Zucchini Noodles with Pesto → Spaghetti Squash with Pesto:**

- Swap zucchini noodles with cooked spaghetti squash.
- Ensure the pesto is gluten-free or make your own with gluten-free ingredients.

3. **Garlic Roasted Brussels Sprouts → Garlic Roasted Carrots**:
- Substitute Brussels sprouts with carrot sticks.
- Follow the same seasoning and roasting instructions.

Dairy-Free Substitutions:

Dairy-free alternatives can be used to create creamy and flavorful dishes without the use of traditional dairy products:

1. **Coconut Yogurt → Dairy-Free Yogurt:**

- Replace dairy yogurt with coconut yogurt or almond milk yogurt.

2. Mashed Root Vegetables → Dairy-Free Mashed Potatoes:

- Use dairy-free milk (such as almond milk or oat milk) instead of regular milk.
- Substitute dairy-free butter or olive oil for butter.

3. Creamy Vegetable Soups → Dairy-Free Creamy Soups:

- Use coconut milk or cashew cream as a dairy-free alternative to heavy cream.
- Blend until smooth for a creamy texture.

Adapting recipes for special diets doesn't have to be complicated or boring. With a little creativity and the right substitutions, you can enjoy a wide variety of flavorful and satisfying meals that cater to your specific dietary needs.

Whether you're vegan, vegetarian, gluten-free, or dairy-free, there's a variety of delicious options you can try.

Conclusion

As you close this chapter, it's essential to reflect on the valuable principles of the SIBO diet that you have learned and how they can positively impact your health and well-being. Let's recap some of the key principles that make the SIBO diet an effective approach to managing Small Intestinal Bacterial Overgrowth:

1. **Low-FODMAP Foods**: By focusing on low-FODMAP foods, you can reduce symptoms like bloating, gas, and abdominal pain commonly associated with SIBO.

2. **Gut-Friendly Foods**: Incorporating fermented foods, bone broth, and gut-healing ingredients can support a

healthy gut microbiome and aid in digestion.

3. **Balanced Nutrition**: Emphasizing a balanced intake of proteins, healthy fats, and carbohydrates ensures you're getting the essential nutrients your body needs.

4. **Personalized Approach**: Adapting recipes to meet your specific dietary needs ensures that you can enjoy delicious meals while following the SIBO diet successfully.

Encouragement and Support for Your Journey:

Embarking on a dietary journey to manage SIBO can sometimes feel overwhelming, but remember, you're not alone. With patience, persistence, and a positive mindset, you can navigate this path successfully and experience improvements in your digestive health and overall well-being.

Here are some words of encouragement to support you along the way:

- Continue to educate yourself about the SIBO diet and stay updated on the latest research and recommendations.

- Pay attention to how your body responds to different foods and adjust your diet accordingly to find what works best for you.

- Connect with healthcare professionals, nutritionists, and support groups who can provide guidance, encouragement, and motivation throughout your journey.

- Celebrate your progress, no matter how small, and remember that every step forward is a step towards better health.

In closing, remember that managing requires patience, dedication, and a willingness to adapt and learn along the way. By embracing the principles of the SIBO diet and incorporating the delicious and nutritious recipes from this cookbook, you're taking proactive steps towards improving your digestive health and overall quality of life.

Thank you for joining us on this culinary adventure, and we wish you success, health, and happiness on your SIBO diet journey. Happy cooking and cheers to a healthier you!

Glossary of Terms

1. **SIBO (Small Intestinal Bacterial Overgrowth)**: A condition characterized by an overgrowth of bacteria in the small intestine, leading to various digestive symptoms.

2. **FODMAPs (Fermentable Oligosaccharides, Disaccharides, Monosaccharides, and Polyols):** A group of carbohydrates that are poorly absorbed in the small intestine and can exacerbate symptoms of SIBO.

3. **Probiotics**: Beneficial bacteria that can help restore balance to the gut microbiome and support digestive health.

4. **Prebiotics**: Non-digestible fibers that feed and nourish the beneficial bacteria in the gut.

5. **Fermentation**: The process by which beneficial bacteria break down sugars and starches, producing beneficial by-products like lactic acid.

6. **Low-FODMAP Diet**: A dietary approach that restricts high-FODMAP foods to manage symptoms of digestive disorders like SIBO.

7. **Gluten-Free**: A diet that excludes gluten, a protein found in wheat, barley, and rye, suitable for individuals with gluten sensitivities or celiac disease.

8. **Dairy-Free**: A diet that excludes dairy products, suitable for

individuals with lactose intolerance or dairy allergies.

This glossary serves as a handy reference guide to help you better understand the terminology used throughout the cookbook and in discussions about the SIBO diet and digestive health.

www.ingramcontent.com/pod-product-compliance
Lightning Source LLC
Chambersburg PA
CBHW061055250726
48653CB00001B/420